COMPLETE GUIDE TO UNDERSTANDING PROSTATECTOMY

Comprehensive Insights, Recovery Tips, Post-Surgery Care, And Lifestyle Adjustments For Optimal Health

KLEIN HOYLE

© [KLEIN HOYLE] [2024]

All rights reserved.

No part of this book may be reproduced, distributed, or transmitted in any form or by any means, including photocopying, recording, or other electronic or mechanical methods, without the publisher's prior written permission, with the exception of brief quotations in critical reviews and certain other noncommercial uses permitted by copyright law.

Disclaimer

The content in this book is based on the author's expertise and comprehension of the topic. The author has no affiliation or link with any corporation, business, or person. This book is meant to give general information and educational material only, and it should not be interpreted as professional medical advice. Always seek the advice of a skilled healthcare expert if you have any queries about medical issues or treatments. The author and publisher expressly disclaim any responsibility resulting directly or indirectly from the use or use of the information included in this book.

Table of Contents

CHAPTER 1 13
- Introduction To Prostatectomy 13
- Understanding The Prostate Gland 13
- Overview Of Prostatectomy 13
- Types Of Prostatectomy Procedures 14
  - 1. Open Prostatectomy: 14
  - 2. Robotic-Assisted Laparoscopic Prostatectomy: 14
  - 3. Laparoscopic Prostatectomy: 15
- Importance Of Prostatectomy In Treating Prostate Cancer 15

CHAPTER 2 17
- Anatomy Of The Prostate Gland 17
- Structure And Function Of The Prostate Gland .17
- The Role Of The Prostate Gland In The Male Reproductive System 18
- Common Prostate Conditions 18
- How Prostate Cancer Develops 19

CHAPTER 3 21
- Preparation For Prostatectomy 21
- Consultation With Healthcare Professionals 21

Pre-Operative Tests And Evaluations 22

Lifestyle Changes Before Surgery 23

Mental And Emotional Preparedness For Procedure 25

CHAPTER 4 27

Types Of Prostatectomy Procedures 27

Radical Prostatectomy 27

Robot-Assisted Laparoscopic Prostatectomy (RALP) 29

Open Prostatectomy 31

Transurethral Resection Of Prostate (TURP) 32

CHAPTER 5 35

Surgical Procedure For Prostatectomy 35

Anesthesia Administration 35

Incision Placement And Procedure Steps 36

Removal Of The Prostate Gland 37

Potential Complications During Surgery 39

CHAPTER 6 43

Recovery And Rehabilitation Post 43

Post-Operative Care Instructions 43

Managing Pain And Discomfort 45

Possible Side Effects And Complications..........46

Timeline For Recovery And Returning To Normal Activities 47

CHAPTER 7 51

Managing Side Effects 51

Bowel Alterations 54

Coping With Side Effects 55

CHAPTER 8 57

Follow-Up Care And Monitoring 57

Scheduled Follow-Up Appointments 57

Monitoring PSA Levels 58

Long-Term Effects Of Prostatectomy 60

Adjustments To Lifestyle And Healthcare Routine 61

CHAPTER 9 65

Alternative Treatments And Therapies 65

Active Surveillance..65

Radiation Treatment Options 66

Hormone Therapy 68

Integrated Approaches To Supporting Prostate Health 69

CHAPTER 10 71
   Life Following Prostatectomy 71
   Emotional Adjustments After Surgery 71
   Maintaining Overall Health And Wellbeing 72
   The Need For Regular Screenings And Check-Ups
   74
   Support Resources For Prostate Cancer Survivors
   75
   Conclusion 77
THE END 80

ABOUT THIS BOOK

"Complete Guide to Understanding Prostatectomy" is a thorough book that will give useful insights into one of the most important operations for treating prostate cancer. With an interesting and educational tone, this book dives into all aspects of prostatectomy, ensuring that readers have a complete idea of what to anticipate before, during, and after the procedure.

Chapter 1 provides the basis by explaining the nuances of prostatectomy. This chapter provides an important primer on the importance of prostatectomy in the treatment of prostate cancer, covering everything from the architecture of the prostate gland to the many kinds of operations accessible. It provides a strong basis for readers to understand the significance of this surgical operation in managing the condition successfully.

Moving on to Chapter 2, readers will be taken on a thorough examination of the anatomy of the prostate gland. This chapter provides readers with the information they need to understand common prostate disorders as well as the development of prostate cancer by explaining its anatomy, function, and role in the male reproductive system. It is an important step toward understanding why prostatectomy is chosen as a therapeutic option.

Chapter 3 goes into the preliminary phase of prostatectomy, highlighting the significance of careful consultation with healthcare providers, pre-operative diagnostics, and lifestyle changes. This chapter addresses the mental and emotional components of preparation, ensuring that readers approach the process with confidence and resilience.

The next chapters dig into the complexities of the surgical process, including several kinds of prostatectomy procedures, anesthetic administration, incision location, and probable problems during operation. Chapters 6 and 7 give detailed insights into the healing and rehabilitation phases, as well as how to control side effects, providing patients with practical advice for navigating the postoperative period.

Chapter 8 emphasizes the necessity of follow-up treatment and monitoring, emphasizing the need for regular checkups and long-term awareness while monitoring PSA levels. Chapter 9 also introduces readers to other treatments and therapies, extending their comprehension of the possibilities accessible to them outside of surgery.

Finally, Chapter 10 provides insight into life following prostatectomy, including emotional adaptations, preserving general health and well-being, and finding support options for prostate cancer survivors. This chapter encourages readers to embrace life with fresh vigor and hope by presenting a comprehensive view of the road after surgery.

In essence, "Complete Guide to Understanding Prostatectomy" serves as an important companion for patients, caregivers, and healthcare professionals alike, providing a wealth of information, advice, and support at every step of the prostate cancer treatment path.

CHAPTER 1

Introduction To Prostatectomy

Understanding The Prostate Gland

The prostate gland, which is sometimes compared to the size of a walnut, is an essential component of the male reproductive system. It is located right below the bladder and surrounds the urethra. It is responsible for the creation of seminal fluid, which nourishes and transports sperm during ejaculation. The prostate gland is vulnerable to a variety of disorders, the most common of which is prostate cancer.

Overview Of Prostatectomy

Prostatectomy is a surgical treatment that removes part or all of the prostate gland. It is generally used to treat prostate cancer, although it may also be used in instances of benign prostatic hyperplasia (BPH), in which the gland enlarges and produces urinary problems. The primary goal of prostatectomy is to remove malignant cells while maintaining urinary function and reducing the risk of complications.

Types Of Prostatectomy Procedures

There are various ways to do a prostatectomy, each with its benefits and considerations:

1. Open Prostatectomy: This classic procedure includes making a single major incision in the lower abdomen to reach and remove the prostate gland. While it allows direct access to the prostate, it often has a lengthier recovery time than other methods.

2. Robotic-Assisted Laparoscopic Prostatectomy: In this minimally invasive operation, a surgeon directs robotic arms carrying specialized tools via tiny incisions in the abdomen. In comparison to open surgery, this method provides greater accuracy and quicker recovery periods.

3. Laparoscopic Prostatectomy: Laparoscopic surgery, like robotic-assisted laparoscopic prostatectomy, uses tiny incisions and a camera to remove the prostate gland. While it may not be as precise as robotic help, it can give advantages such as less discomfort and faster recovery.

4. Transurethral Resection of the Prostate (TURP) is generally used to treat benign prostatic hyperplasia (BPH), not prostate cancer. It entails placing a specialized device into the urethra to remove excessive prostate tissue that is causing urinary blockage. While TURP is less invasive than other prostatectomy techniques, it is not recommended for cancer therapy.

Importance Of Prostatectomy In Treating Prostate Cancer

Prostatectomy is essential in the treatment of prostate cancer, particularly when the disease is confined inside the prostate gland. Prostatectomy, which removes malignant tissue, tries to destroy cancer cells and prevent the illness from spreading to other areas of the body. Furthermore, prostatectomy may help relieve symptoms like trouble peeing or frequent urination, hence enhancing the patient's quality of life.

Understanding the different kinds of prostatectomy procedures and their benefits enables patients and healthcare professionals to make more educated judgments about treatment alternatives. While prostatectomy is a significant surgical surgery, advances in surgical methods and technology have resulted in better results and lower risks for people receiving this therapy for prostate cancer.

CHAPTER 2

Anatomy Of The Prostate Gland

Structure And Function Of The Prostate Gland

The prostate gland is a vital component of the male reproductive system that is sometimes equated to the size of a walnut. It is located slightly below the bladder and in front of the rectum, and it surrounds the urethra, the tube that transports urine and sperm from the body. The prostate glands main purpose is to create seminal fluid, a milky liquid that nourishes and transports sperm after ejaculation.

The gland is made up of three kinds of tissue: glandular tissue, which produces seminal fluid, fibromuscular tissue, which provides structural support, and smooth muscle tissue, which aids in the evacuation of semen during ejaculation.

This complicated composition guarantees the gland's appropriate activity throughout the reproductive process.

The Role Of The Prostate Gland In The Male Reproductive System

Male fertility and sexual function are heavily dependent on the prostate gland. During ejaculation, muscles in the prostate gland flex to release seminal fluid into the urethra, where it combines with sperm from the testes and other fluids from accessory glands to produce semen. This process, known as emission, is necessary for the movement and viability of sperm.

Furthermore, the prostate gland produces prostate-specific antigen (PSA), an enzyme that liquefies semen after ejaculation, hence improving sperm motility. This function is critical to proper fertilization and conception.

Common Prostate Conditions

Several disorders may affect the prostate gland, resulting in a variety of symptoms and problems. Benign prostatic hyperplasia (BPH) is a non-cancerous growth of the prostate gland that often causes urinary symptoms such as frequent urination, difficulty initiating or halting urine flow, and incomplete bladder emptying.

Prostatitis, or inflammation of the prostate gland, may be caused by a bacterial infection or other factors, resulting in pelvic discomfort, urine issues, and sexual dysfunction. Prostate cancer, the most prevalent disease in males, develops when abnormal cells in the prostate gland expand rapidly, developing tumors that may spread to other areas of the body if not treated.

How Prostate Cancer Develops

Prostate cancer often starts with tiny alterations in the prostate gland's cells, which are frequently unnoticed without medical intervention. Over time, these aberrant cells may develop a tiny tumor inside the gland, initially limited to the prostate tissue (localized prostate cancer).

As the cancer grows, it may spread to neighboring tissues and organs, including the seminal vesicles, bladder, and rectum. In advanced stages, prostate cancer may spread to distant areas in the body, such as the bones, lymph nodes, or other organs, affecting prognosis and treatment choices substantially.

Understanding the anatomy of the prostate gland, its role in the male reproductive system, common prostate conditions, and the progression of prostate cancer is critical for gaining a comprehensive understanding of prostate health and the various treatment options available for prostate-related issues.

CHAPTER 3

Preparation For Prostatectomy

Consultation With Healthcare Professionals

Before having a prostatectomy, it is essential to have extensive discussions with healthcare specialists. These consultations usually include conversations with a urologist, who specializes in the urinary tract and male reproductive systems. During these appointments, the urologist will evaluate your medical history, present health, and the details of your prostate disease.

The consultation serves several goals. First and foremost, it enables the urologist to decide if a prostatectomy is the best therapeutic choice for your problem.

They will go over the process in detail, including the possible risks and advantages, as well as any alternative therapies that may be available.

Additionally, the consultation allows you to ask questions and voice any concerns you may have regarding the operation. It is important to be open and honest throughout these talks so that you completely understand what to anticipate before, during, and after surgery.

Pre-Operative Tests And Evaluations

Various pre-operative tests and assessments will be performed to check your general health and determine your suitability for surgery. These tests may include:

• Blood tests will assess general health, including blood cell count, and kidney and liver function.

• Urine samples may be tested for symptoms of infection or urinary tract abnormalities.

- Imaging studies (e.g., ultrasound, MRI, CT scans) may assess prostate gland size and location, as well as detect cancer spread to adjacent tissues.

- An electrocardiogram (ECG) may examine your heart's electrical activity and identify potential dangers during operation.

- A physical examination will evaluate your overall health, vital signs, pulmonary function, and fitness for surgery.

These tests assist the surgical team in gathering critical information about your health condition and any possible concerns that must be addressed before starting with the prostatectomy.

Lifestyle Changes Before Surgery

Making lifestyle changes before having a prostatectomy will help you enhance your overall health and recovery results. Common modifications may include:

- Quit smoking to improve post-surgery healing and reduce problems. Quitting smoking before surgery may improve circulation, lower the chance of infection, and speed up recovery.

- Eating a balanced diet with fruits, vegetables, lean meats, and whole grains helps promote healing and immunological function. Staying hydrated is also crucial, so drink lots of water.

- Regular physical exercise improves cardiovascular health, muscular strength, and general well-being. However, before beginning any new workout plan, you must contact your healthcare professional, particularly if you have pre-existing health concerns.

- Managing stress: Stress may hinder the body's healing process and lead to issues. Relaxation practices such as deep breathing, meditation, and yoga may help decrease stress and develop a good attitude before surgery.

By adopting these lifestyle changes, you may better prepare your body and mind for the forthcoming prostatectomy and improve your overall recovery.

Mental And Emotional Preparedness For Procedure

Preparing psychologically and emotionally for a prostatectomy is as vital as preparing physically. Surgery may be stressful and anxiety-inducing, but there are things you can do to manage these feelings and feel better prepared:

- Educate yourself about the prostatectomy process and what to anticipate before, during, and after surgery. Understanding the procedure might assist in reducing concerns and anxieties.

- Reach out to friends, relatives, or support groups who have had similar treatments. Hearing about their experiences, as well as getting encouragement and support, may make you feel less alone and better prepared for the challenges ahead.

• Express your emotions: It's natural to have dread, anxiety, and grief before surgery. Don't be afraid to communicate these emotions to your healthcare staff or loved ones. They can provide comfort, support, and advice to help you manage.

• Incorporate relaxation methods into your everyday routine to reduce stress and anxiety. Deep breathing, gradual muscle relaxation, and guided visualization are all techniques that may help you feel more relaxed and at ease.

• Stay positive: Highlight the benefits of the operation, such as increased health and quality of life. Maintaining a good attitude will allow you to face the process with confidence and perseverance.

CHAPTER 4

Types Of Prostatectomy Procedures

Radical Prostatectomy

Radical prostatectomy is a surgical treatment that is often performed to treat prostate cancer. The whole prostate gland, as well as surrounding tissues such as seminal vesicles and lymph nodes, are removed. This surgery seeks to remove malignant cells and prevent cancer from spreading to other regions of the body.

Before surgery, the patient is subjected to a series of tests and examinations to establish the stage and extent of the malignancy. These may involve imaging tests such as MRIs or CT scans, as well as biopsies to confirm the presence of cancer cells in the prostate.

During surgery, the patient is given general anesthesia to ensure that they remain asleep and painless during the process.

Depending on the surgical method, the surgeon will create an incision in the lower abdomen or between the anus and scrotum.

A radical retropubic prostatectomy involves making an incision in the lower abdomen. A radical perineal prostatectomy involves making an incision between the anus and the scrotum. The size and location of the tumor, as well as the surgeon's competence, all influence the strategy used.

Once the prostate gland is uncovered, the surgeon gently removes it and the surrounding tissues. The nerves and blood arteries that control erectile function and urine continence are carefully preserved.

After removing the prostate, the surgeon gently seals the incision and inserts a drainage tube to remove any extra fluid or blood from the surgical site. The patient is subsequently transferred to the recovery room and carefully monitored for problems.

Recovery following a radical prostatectomy might take weeks or months, depending on the person and the amount of the operation. Patients should avoid heavy lifting and vigorous exercise during this period and adhere to their doctor's instructions for medication and follow-up sessions.

Robot-Assisted Laparoscopic Prostatectomy (RALP)

Robot-assisted laparoscopic prostatectomy (RALP) is a minimally invasive surgical procedure used to remove the prostate. It combines the precision of laparoscopic surgery with the dexterity of robotic technology to improve the procedure's accuracy and control.

RALP involves the surgeon making numerous tiny incisions in the belly through which specialized tools and a camera are introduced. The surgeon controls this equipment from a console in the operating room, allowing them to operate the robotic arms with accuracy.

The robotic device gives a three-dimensional image of the surgical site, enabling the physician to see more clearly and accurately than conventional laparoscopic surgery. This improves the surgeon's ability to remove the prostate gland while causing little injury to surrounding tissues.

One of the primary benefits of RALP is its minimally invasive nature, which leads to smaller incisions, less blood loss, and quicker recovery periods than open surgery. Patients who undergo RALP often suffer less discomfort and scarring, as well as a shorter hospital stay.

Despite its advantages, RALP may not be appropriate for all patients, particularly those with significant scarring from prior procedures or certain anatomical variances.

Patients should examine their choices with their surgeon to identify the best treatment approach for their specific requirements.

Open Prostatectomy

Open prostatectomy is a classic surgical procedure for removing the prostate gland. It entails creating a single big incision in the lower abdomen to reach and remove the prostate gland.

During the surgery, the surgeon meticulously dissects the tissues that surround the prostate gland to expose it completely. The prostate gland is then removed, along with any nearby tissues that may contain cancer cells.

Open prostatectomy is usually conducted under general anesthesia to keep the patient asleep and pain-free during the surgery. When feasible, the surgeon may utilize nerve-sparing procedures to maintain the nerves that control erectile function and urine continence.

After removing the prostate gland, the surgeon gently seals the incision and inserts a drainage tube to remove any excess fluid or blood from the operative area. The patient is subsequently transferred to the recovery room and carefully monitored for problems.

Recovery following an open prostatectomy might take several weeks to months, depending on the person and the scope of the procedure. Patients should avoid heavy lifting and vigorous exercise during this period and adhere to their doctor's instructions for medication and follow-up sessions.

Transurethral Resection Of Prostate (TURP)

Transurethral resection of the prostate (TURP) is a minimally invasive surgical treatment used to treat benign prostatic hyperplasia (BPH), which is a non-cancerous expansion of the prostate gland. It is conducted using a resectoscope, which is introduced into the urethra and directed to the prostate gland.

During TURP, the surgeon uses the resectoscope to remove extra prostate tissue that is obstructing the urethra and producing urinary problems. This is accomplished by delivering an electric current via a wire loop connected to the resectoscope, cutting away extra tissue and cauterizing any bleeding.

TURP is usually conducted using spinal or general anesthesia to keep the patient comfortable and pain-free during the surgery. The surgeon may also use a continuous irrigation device to cleanse the bladder and remove any tissue pieces or blood.

One of the primary benefits of TURP is that it is less intrusive than open surgery, resulting in quicker recovery periods and a lower risk of complications. However, TURP may not be appropriate for many individuals, particularly those with big prostates or certain medical problems.

Following the surgery, the patient is carefully observed in the recovery area and may be returned home on the same day or after a brief hospitalization. To ensure a smooth recovery, patients should follow their doctor's post-operative care recommendations, which include medication and follow-up sessions.

CHAPTER 5

Surgical Procedure For Prostatectomy

Anesthesia Administration

Anesthesia administration is an important stage in the surgical process of prostatectomy, ensuring that the patient is comfortable and pain-free during the treatment. Before the operation, the anesthesia team will review the patient's medical history, current medicines, and general health to select the best kind and amount of anesthetic.

In most prostatectomy operations, two forms of anesthesia are used: general anesthesia and regional anesthesia. General anesthesia is the use of drugs to produce unconsciousness, enabling the patient to sleep and be ignorant of the procedure. Regional anesthesia, on the other hand, entails numbing particular areas of the body, such as the lower half, using local anesthetic.

Once the kind of anesthetic has been determined, the anesthesia team will deliver it by intravenous injection or inhalation, depending on the patient's health and the surgical team's preferences. Throughout the surgery, the anesthesia team will carefully monitor the patient's vital signs to guarantee their safety and comfort.

Incision Placement And Procedure Steps

The incision location and procedural phases in prostatectomy procedures may differ based on the method employed, such as open, laparoscopic, or robotic-assisted surgery. The primary objective, however, remains the same: to remove the prostate gland safely and effectively while causing as little harm as possible to surrounding tissues and organs.

An open prostatectomy involves making a single big incision in the lower abdomen, which allows the surgeon direct access to the prostate gland. The surrounding tissues and muscles may be gently pushed aside to reveal the prostate. Once the prostate is exposed, the surgeon delicately removes it while protecting adjacent nerves and blood arteries that are essential for urine and sexual function.

During laparoscopic and robotic-assisted prostatectomy, numerous small incisions are made in the abdomen to introduce specialized devices and a tiny camera. This equipment enables the surgeon to do the treatment with more accuracy and control by using the enlarged pictures offered by the camera. The prostate is subsequently dissected and removed using these devices, which follow the same stages as open surgery but with smaller incisions and less tissue damage.

Throughout the treatment, the surgical team will collaborate to ensure that each step is carried out safely and effectively, reducing the risk of problems and improving the patient's prognosis.

Removal Of The Prostate Gland

The surgical procedure centers on the removal of the prostate gland, often known as prostatectomy. Whether open, laparoscopic, or robotic-assisted, the main goal is to thoroughly remove the prostate while preserving urinary and sexual function as much as feasible.

During the treatment, the surgeon gently dissects the prostate gland away from surrounding tissues and organs, taking care not to harm neighboring nerves and blood arteries that are essential for urine control and sexual function. Once the prostate is free of its attachments, it is gently removed from the body via the surgical incision(s).

In certain circumstances, especially if prostate cancer is confined and low-risk, the surgeon may choose a nerve-sparing method, which seeks to save the nerves that control erectile function. To minimize nerve injury when removing the prostate, this method demands painstaking dissection and accuracy.

After the prostate gland is removed, the surgical team will thoroughly evaluate the surgical site for any symptoms of bleeding or other issues before closing the incisions and completing the treatment. Postoperative care and recuperation will next commence, with the patient constantly watched for symptoms of problems and given appropriate pain relief and support.

Potential Complications During Surgery

Despite advances in surgical procedures and technology, prostatectomy operations include inherent risks of consequences, which may range from mild to serious. These difficulties may occur for a variety of reasons, including the patient's general health, the difficulty of the operation, and unanticipated anatomical variances.

Excessive bleeding during prostatectomy surgery is a possible complication that may develop as a result of blood vessel injury or poor hemostasis. To reduce this danger, the surgical team uses precise surgical techniques, such as thorough dissection and the use of specialist devices to seal blood veins.

Another potential risk is injury to neighboring tissues, such as the urinary sphincter or adjoining nerves, which might result in urine incontinence or erectile dysfunction. To reduce these dangers, surgeons get significant training and use nerve-sparing procedures wherever possible, which preserve key anatomical structures while removing the prostate.

Infection is also a worry after prostatectomy surgery since the surgical site is prone to bacterial contamination. To mitigate this risk, patients are often given antibiotics before and after surgery, and rigorous sterile measures are used during the process.

Other potential problems include urine retention, blood clots, and anesthesia-related disorders, all of which are thoroughly monitored and controlled by the surgical team to guarantee the patient's best result.

Despite these possible hazards, the advantages of prostatectomy in treating prostate cancer frequently exceed the risks, especially when done by competent surgeons at specialized clinics that provide multidisciplinary care.

CHAPTER 6

Recovery And Rehabilitation Post

Post-Operative Care Instructions

Following a prostatectomy, your post-operative care is critical for a successful recovery. Your healthcare staff will give you particular recommendations based on your situation, but here are some broad guidelines to anticipate.

First and foremost, you must adhere to your doctor's wound care guidelines. Depending on the kind of surgery you had (open, laparoscopic, or robotic-assisted), you may have incisions that need care. Keep the incision clean and dry, and follow any dressing changes recommended by your healthcare practitioner. They may also advise on first shower and bathing limitations.

Additionally, your healthcare staff will most likely suggest progressively increasing physical exercise. While it is important to relax and allow your body to recover, mild walking and moderate motions help improve circulation and avoid blood clots. However, you should avoid vigorous activity or heavy lifting until your doctor clears you, which is normally approximately six weeks after surgery.

You'll also get tips on nutrition and hydration. Staying hydrated and eating a well-balanced diet is vital for your body's recuperation. Your doctor may advise you to make dietary changes to avoid constipation or bladder discomfort while you recuperate.

Finally, follow-up visits with your healthcare professional are critical. These sessions enable your doctor to monitor your progress, discuss any concerns or issues, and make changes to your treatment plan as necessary.

Managing Pain And Discomfort

Pain management is an important part of post-prostatectomy rehabilitation. Your healthcare provider will prescribe pain medication to help you feel better throughout the early stages of recovery. To get the best pain relief, use these drugs exactly as prescribed.

In addition to medicine, you may use alternative methods to control pain and discomfort. Applying cold packs to the surgery site helps decrease swelling and numb it, offering comfort. However, be sure to follow your doctor's advice for the length and frequency of ice pack usage.

Furthermore, adopting relaxation methods such as deep breathing exercises or meditation might aid in pain relief and general well-being. Listen to your body and rest as required, but also integrate light movement and activities to avoid stiffness and encourage recovery.

If you are experiencing chronic or increasing pain despite medication and home treatments, contact your healthcare professional right once. They may evaluate your situation and modify your pain management strategy appropriately.

Possible Side Effects And Complications

While prostatectomy is typically safe, it, like any other surgical operation, has the possibility of problems. Understanding these dangers might help you identify warning signals and seek immediate medical assistance if required.

Urinary incontinence and erectile dysfunction are among the most prevalent adverse effects after prostatectomy. These side effects might differ based on the kind of surgery done and personal characteristics such as age and general health. Your healthcare team will discuss these possible side effects with you before surgery and provide post-operative management measures.

In addition to urinary and sexual side effects, infection, blood clots, and tissue harm are also possible risks. Fever, redness, or discharge at the incision site are all markers of infection, and you should tell your healthcare practitioner if you suffer any of these symptoms.

Blood clots are another possible consequence after surgery. A blood clot may cause swelling, discomfort, or redness in the legs. If you encounter any of these symptoms, get medical treatment right once, since blood clots may be fatal if not treated quickly.

Timeline For Recovery And Returning To Normal Activities

The recovery period after a prostatectomy varies based on various variables, including the kind of surgery done, individual healing capabilities, and any issues that arise throughout the recovery process. However, here's a basic idea of what to expect:

- During the first several days after surgery, you may suffer pain and should rest and gradually begin mild activities as tolerated.

- During the first few weeks after surgery, gradually raise your activity level while watching for potential consequences including infection or blood clots. Your doctor may offer pelvic floor exercises to help you restore bladder control.

- Within the first few months, patients often have improved urine control and may resume more rigorous activities like exercise or lifting. However, you must continue to follow your doctor's advice and attend follow-up consultations.

- Prostatectomy recovery might take months or even years. While certain adverse effects, such as urine incontinence or erectile dysfunction, may remain, many patients can return to regular activities and have a high quality of life after surgery.

It is important to be patient with yourself throughout the healing process and allow your body the time it needs to heal completely. Your healthcare staff is available to help you every step of the journey and may provide advice and assistance as required.

CHAPTER 7

Managing Side Effects

Urinary incontinence, or the involuntary flow of pee, is a typical adverse effect after prostatectomy. This happens because the procedure may harm the muscles and nerves that regulate bladder function. It's important to note that, although this might be upsetting, it's usually transient and improves with time as the body adapts.

Pelvic floor muscle exercises, or Kegel exercises, are one method for treating urine incontinence. These exercises help strengthen the muscles that govern urine, resulting in improved bladder control. Your healthcare physician or physical therapist can help you do these exercises appropriately.

In addition to exercise, lifestyle changes may aid with urine incontinence. Avoiding coffee and alcohol, which may irritate the bladder, as well as keeping a healthy weight, can help to relieve bladder strain. Timed voiding, in which you arrange frequent restroom breaks, may also assist in avoiding accidents.

More severe forms of urine incontinence may be treated medically. These might include drugs to alleviate bladder spasms or surgical techniques such as placing a sling to support the bladder neck. It is important to examine these alternatives with your healthcare physician to identify the best course of action for your particular case.

Another possible adverse effect of prostatectomy is erectile dysfunction (ED), which is the inability to attain or maintain a satisfactory erection for sexual intercourse. This happens because the procedure may harm the nerves and blood vessels that trigger erections.

It's crucial to understand that, although eating disorders may be difficult to manage, there are numerous treatment options accessible.

Oral drugs such as sildenafil (Viagra), tadalafil (Cialis), and vardenafil (Levitra) increase blood flow to the penis, allowing for erections.

Other treatments for erectile dysfunction include vacuum erection devices, which utilize suction to pull blood into the penis, and penile implants, which are surgically implanted devices that allow for on-demand erections. Counseling or sex therapy may also help address any psychological aspects that contribute to eating disorders.

It is important to communicate openly and honestly with your healthcare physician about any issues or problems you may be having with erectile function. They can help you navigate the different treatment choices and create a plan that is specific to your requirements and interests.

Bowel Alterations

Because of the prostate's proximity to the rectum and the effects of the operation on bowel function, bowel alterations such as diarrhea or constipation may develop after prostatectomy. These alterations are usually transitory and gradually improve as the body recovers.

Dietary alterations are one technique for treating gastrointestinal changes. Consuming more fiber may help regulate bowel movements and prevent constipation, while avoiding items that might aggravate diarrhea, such as spicy or oily meals, can help reduce symptoms.

In addition to dietary adjustments, medicines may be administered to alleviate gastrointestinal symptoms. Anti-diarrheal drugs, for example, may reduce diarrhea, whilst stool softeners or laxatives can aid with constipation. To identify the best course of action for any gastrointestinal symptoms you may be experiencing, consult with your healthcare physician.

Coping With Side Effects

Coping with the side effects of a prostatectomy may be difficult, but some ways can help make the process more tolerable. Education and comprehension are critical components. Learning about the possible side effects of surgery ahead of time can help you psychologically and emotionally prepare for what to anticipate.

Support from loved ones and healthcare experts may also be quite beneficial at this time. Don't be afraid to seek out friends, family, or support groups for emotional help and encouragement. Your healthcare professional may also help you manage side effects and adapt to life following surgery.

Furthermore, leading a healthy lifestyle may boost general well-being and aid in healing. This involves eating a well-balanced diet, being physically active within the limits of your recovery, and obtaining enough relaxation and sleep.

Finally, it's important to maintain reasonable expectations and be patient with yourself as you go through the rehabilitation process. Healing takes time, and it is natural to have highs and lows along the road. By taking things one day at a time and concentrating on self-care, you may gradually adapt to life after prostatectomy while reducing the burden of side effects on your quality of life.

CHAPTER 8

Follow-Up Care And Monitoring

Scheduled Follow-Up Appointments

Following a prostatectomy, it is important to schedule frequent follow-up sessions to assess your healing status and handle any potential issues as soon as possible. These visits are usually planned at regular intervals in the months after your operation. During these appointments, your healthcare professional will evaluate your general health, track your recovery, and answer any concerns or questions you may have.

At your follow-up consultations, your healthcare practitioner will do a physical examination to look for any symptoms of problems, such as infection or unusual healing. They may also request further tests, such as blood work or imaging scans, to assess the health of your prostate and surrounding tissues.

These sessions also allow you to address any changes in your symptoms or concerns regarding your rehabilitation. Your healthcare practitioner may advise you on how to manage any residual surgery-related side effects and provide suggestions to help you recuperate faster.

It is important to attend all planned follow-up visits as directed by your healthcare practitioner to ensure that you get the treatment and support you need during your recovery.

Monitoring PSA Levels

Monitoring prostate-specific antigen (PSA) levels after a prostatectomy is an important element of post-operative treatment. PSA is a protein generated by the prostate gland, and high levels might suggest prostate cancer or other prostate-related disorders.

PSA values usually drop dramatically following prostate removal surgery. Monitoring PSA levels throughout time enables healthcare practitioners to identify any possible return of prostate cancer or other issues early on.

PSA testing is often conducted at regular intervals after prostatectomy, with the frequency chosen by your healthcare physician depending on your specific risk factors and medical history. In certain situations, PSA levels may be undetectable following surgery, suggesting a favorable result. However, a growing PSA result may need further testing, like as imaging scans or biopsies, to rule out recurring illness.

It is critical that you discuss the importance of PSA monitoring with your healthcare physician and follow the suggested testing regimen. PSA levels should be monitored regularly to guarantee early diagnosis and treatment of any recurring prostate cancer or other prostate-related disorders.

Long-Term Effects Of Prostatectomy

While prostatectomy helps treat prostate cancer, surgery may have long-term consequences for a person's health and quality of life. Understanding these possible consequences might assist patients in better preparing for life after surgery and making educated choices regarding their post-surgical care.

Erectile dysfunction (ED) is a frequent long-term side effect of prostatectomy, which may be caused by injury to the nerves and blood vessels that control erections. While some men may develop acute ED after surgery, others may have ongoing or chronic problems. Fortunately, there are many therapy options for erectile dysfunction, including oral drugs, vacuum erection devices, penile injections, and surgical implants.

Another possible long-term side effect of prostatectomy is urine incontinence, which may arise as a result of injury to the urethral sphincter or other urinary control structures. While many men's urine continence improves with time, others may still have leakage or urgency. Pelvic floor exercises, lifestyle changes, and, in certain situations, surgical procedures may all help treat urine incontinence and improve bladder control.

In addition to physical repercussions, prostatectomy may have emotional and psychological consequences for men and their spouses. Coping with prostate cancer, having surgery, and adapting to changes in sexual function and urine control may be difficult for some people. Seeking assistance from healthcare practitioners, support groups, or mental health specialists may help you navigate these emotional issues and improve your overall well-being.

Adjustments To Lifestyle And Healthcare Routine

Making changes to your lifestyle and healthcare practice after prostatectomy may help you recover more quickly and improve long-term health and wellness. Diet, exercise, medication management, and general self-care habits may all be affected by these changes.

Dietary changes may include adding additional fruits, vegetables, whole grains, and lean meats to your meals to improve general health and recuperation. Some people may benefit from avoiding foods or drinks that irritate the bladder or worsen urinary symptoms.

Regular exercise is critical for maintaining physical fitness, controlling weight, and enhancing general well-being after prostatectomy. Walking, swimming, and cycling may all assist in enhancing your cardiovascular health, muscular strength, and flexibility. It is critical to contact your healthcare professional before beginning any new fitness routine and to gradually increase intensity as tolerated.

Medication management may include taking prescription drugs as indicated to alleviate pain, prevent infection, and handle other postoperative issues. It is critical that you strictly adhere to your healthcare provider's instructions and discuss any side effects or concerns as soon as possible.

In addition to these lifestyle changes, keeping frequent follow-up meetings with your healthcare practitioner and following suggested screening and monitoring protocols is critical for long-term health maintenance. By being proactive about your health and well-being, you may reduce the risk of problems and encourage the best possible results after prostatectomy.

CHAPTER 9

Alternative Treatments And Therapies

Active Surveillance

Active surveillance is a prostate cancer care technique in which the illness is continuously monitored rather than immediately undergoing surgery or other harsh therapies. This method is often suggested for men with low-risk prostate cancer, which is slow-growing and unlikely to cause damage in the near term.

Regular check-ups, including PSA testing, digital rectal examinations, and, in some cases, biopsies, are performed during active surveillance to monitor the cancer's growth. These check-ups assist healthcare experts in determining whether the cancer is progressing and if intervention, such as surgery or radiation treatment, is required.

One of the primary benefits of active monitoring is that it avoids the risks and consequences associated with surgery or radiation treatment. It also helps men to maintain their quality of life while avoiding unneeded therapy if their disease is not advancing.

However, active surveillance necessitates close monitoring and might create anxiety in some men who are concerned about the risk of their disease developing. Men under active surveillance must collaborate actively with their healthcare team to ensure they are getting enough monitoring and assistance.

Radiation Treatment Options

Radiation therapy is a typical treatment for prostate cancer that uses high-energy radiation to destroy cancer cells. There are various radiation treatment alternatives available, including external beam radiation therapy (EBRT) and brachytherapy.

EBRT includes sending radiation beams from outside the body to the prostate gland. This therapy is usually given over a few weeks, with daily treatments lasting a few minutes each. EBRT is non-invasive and may be an effective therapy for localized prostate cancer.

Brachytherapy, commonly known as internal radiation therapy, is placing radioactive seeds directly into the prostate gland. These seeds release radiation, which kills adjacent cancer cells over time. Brachytherapy is a minimally invasive method that may be used as a single treatment or in conjunction with EBRT.

Both EBRT and brachytherapy have equal effectiveness rates in the treatment of prostate cancer, however, the decision between the two is determined by criteria such as disease stage, patient general health, and personal preferences.

Hormone Therapy

Hormone therapy, commonly known as androgen deprivation therapy (ADT), is a prostate cancer treatment strategy that tries to lower the body's levels of male hormones like testosterone. Prostate cancer cells depend on male hormones to develop and spread, therefore lowering hormone levels may halt disease progression.

Hormone treatment may be delivered by injections, oral pills, or surgical removal of the testicles (orchiectomy). It is often used in conjunction with other therapies, such as radiation therapy or chemotherapy, to increase their efficacy.

While hormone treatment may help decrease prostate cancer development, it can also induce adverse effects including hot flashes, loss of libido, erectile dysfunction, and exhaustion. These side effects may have a substantial influence on a man's quality of life, so patients should address them with their doctor before beginning hormone treatment.

Integrated Approaches To Supporting Prostate Health

Integrative approaches to prostate health include lifestyle adjustments, dietary changes, and complementary treatments to assist men with prostate problems manage symptoms and enhance their overall well-being.

Regular exercise, keeping a healthy weight, and refraining from smoking and excessive alcohol intake are all examples of lifestyle changes that may benefit prostate health. Exercise, in particular, has been demonstrated to lower the chance of getting prostate cancer and improve results for men receiving treatment.

Dietary adjustments, such as eating more fruits, vegetables, and whole grains while consuming less red meat and processed foods, may also enhance prostate health. Certain nutrients, including lycopene present in tomatoes, as well as antioxidants such as vitamin E and selenium, have been related to a decreased risk of prostate cancer.

Acupuncture, massage therapy, and yoga are examples of complementary treatments that may help relieve symptoms such as discomfort, exhaustion, and anxiety in men with prostate problems. While these treatments may not directly cure cancer, they can give important support and enhance quality of life during and after treatment.

Men contemplating integrative ways to promote prostate health should contact their healthcare physician to confirm that these tactics are safe and suitable for their specific requirements.

CHAPTER 10

Life Following Prostatectomy

Emotional Adjustments After Surgery

It is normal to have a variety of feelings after a prostatectomy. From relief to worry, everyone's path is unique. Initially, you may be happy that the operation is finished and optimistic about your future health. However, it is normal to feel nervous or even melancholy while you adapt to changes in your body and lifestyle.

One of the most difficult emotional obstacles after surgery is coping with the procedure's probable adverse effects, such as urine incontinence or erectile dysfunction. These challenges may influence your self-esteem and sense of masculinity, leaving you feeling frustrated or depressed.

It's important to realize that these side effects are usually transient and may improve with proper treatment and support.

Getting assistance from loved ones, joining a support group, or seeking therapy may all be quite beneficial during this emotional transition phase. Openly discussing your thoughts and worries with people who have gone through similar circumstances may bring validation and comfort. Furthermore, participating in self-care activities like exercise, meditation, or hobbies may assist decrease stress and enhance your mental well-being.

Maintaining Overall Health And Wellbeing

Maintaining general health and well-being is critical after a prostatectomy. While surgery directly targets malignant cells, maintaining a healthy lifestyle may help lower the chance of cancer recurrence and enhance your quality of life.

Maintaining a healthy diet is one of the most crucial parts of post-surgical recovery. Include lots of fruits, vegetables, healthy grains, and lean proteins in your meals while reducing processed foods, sugary snacks, and excessive red meat. Staying hydrated with enough water is also critical for general health and recovery.

Regular exercise is another important part of a healthy lifestyle after surgery. Walking, swimming, or cycling may all help you gain strength, and stamina, and enhance your mood. Begin cautiously, then gradually increase the intensity and length of your exercises as your body permits.

Getting enough sleep is critical for recovery and general well-being. Aim for seven to nine hours of excellent sleep every night, and create a pleasant bedtime ritual to help you unwind and prepare for sleep.

The Need For Regular Screenings And Check-Ups

Even after a prostatectomy, it is important to maintain frequent screenings and check-ups to monitor your health and identify any possible problems early. Your healthcare practitioner will propose a follow-up plan based on your specific requirements and risk factors.

These screenings may involve routine blood tests to monitor your prostate-specific antigen (PSA) levels, as well as physical examinations and imaging studies if required. Early diagnosis of cancer recurrence or other health issues may greatly enhance treatment effectiveness and results.

In addition to medical tests, it is critical to monitor any changes in your body and quickly report them to your healthcare professional. This includes symptoms including bladder issues, sexual dysfunction, and unexplained pain or discomfort.

Support Resources For Prostate Cancer Survivors

Finding information for prostate cancer survivors may be quite helpful as you navigate life following surgery. Many organizations, support groups, and online communities exist to provide information, education, and emotional support to those impacted by prostate cancer.

These materials may help you learn about treatment choices, managing side effects, and dealing with the emotional problems of a cancer diagnosis. They also allow you to connect with others who understand what you're going through and can give empathy, support, and practical guidance.

Many hospitals and cancer centers provide support programs tailored to prostate cancer survivors, such as counseling services, support groups, and educational courses. Furthermore, internet tools like websites, forums, and social media groups may help you interact with people and obtain knowledge from the comfort of your own home.

By using these tools, you may obtain vital information, get emotional support, and form a feeling of community with people who understand your situation. Remember that you are not alone on this journey, and there are people and resources available to assist you every step of the way.

Conclusion

Finally, both patients and healthcare professionals need a thorough grasp of prostatectomy. This surgical operation, whether done open, laparoscopic, or robotically, is mainly intended to treat prostate cancer. However, it may also be used to treat benign prostatic hyperplasia (BPH) and other prostate-related diseases.

This tutorial has covered many facets of prostatectomy, from the architecture and function of the prostate gland to the complexities of the surgical process itself. We've spoken about the many forms of prostatectomy, their indications, and the risks and consequences that come with each procedure.

We have emphasized the need for patient education and collaborative decision-making in the treatment of prostate cancer. Patients must be well-educated about the various treatment choices, including the possible advantages and risks of prostatectomy, to make informed decisions that are consistent with their preferences and values.

Furthermore, we emphasized the need for a multidisciplinary approach to prostate cancer treatment. Urologists, oncologists, radiologists, and other healthcare specialists must work together to ensure that patients having prostatectomy have the best possible results. From preoperative examination and surgical planning to postoperative care and long-term follow-up, coordinated efforts are required at all stages of the treatment process.

We have also discussed the possible effect of prostatectomy on quality of life, namely urinary and sexual function. While advances in surgical procedures and perioperative care have improved functional results, many patients continue to be concerned about these difficulties. As a result, further research and innovation are required to improve surgical methods and reduce the negative consequences of prostatectomy on patient well-being.

Finally, prostatectomy is an important treatment option for prostate cancer and other prostate-related disorders. By offering a thorough review of this surgical technique, we intend to provide patients with the information they need to actively engage in their care and make educated choices about their treatment options. Furthermore, we want to foster continuing communication and cooperation among healthcare professionals to improve patient outcomes and the quality of care for those undergoing prostatectomy.

THE END

www.ingramcontent.com/pod-product-compliance
Lightning Source LLC
Chambersburg PA
CBHW072017230526
45479CB00008B/216